Introduction

Neck pain is relatively common in t[...] occur as we age. It is estimated that 1[...] perience neck pain at any given time. It accounts for 1% of all patient visits to a primary care physician. The exact cause of the pain varies depending upon the mechanism of injury and structure injured, whether bone, muscle, ligament, or disc. The most common cause of pain is a muscle strain, although other causes include arthritis, disc herniation, ligament sprain, or fracture. The type and severity of symptoms will vary depending on the cause but will commonly lead to pain and loss of motion in the neck region or upper extremity. If not treated appropriately, prolonged injury can lead to greater loss of mobility and function that can impact activities of daily living or one's ability to participate at work.

Fortunately, the most common causes of most acute neck pain are not serious and will improve over a relatively short period of time. Most symptoms may be treated over a several-week period with relative rest, medication, proper stretching, and improved posture. Subsequent symptoms may be prevented by continued stretching and strengthening of the neck muscles. Prolonged or severe symptoms will require further treatment under the guidance of a physician to help prevent disability The goal of this booklet is to describe the common causes of acute neck pain and strategies for the prevention and treatment of such injuries.

Structure (Anatomy) of the Neck

The neck is made up of bones, ligaments, and muscles that connect the head to the rest of the body. It is designed to move the head and protect the spinal cord as it travels to the body. The various components of the neck are shown in Figure 1.

- The neck or cervical spine bones are called vertebrae, which are bones stacked one on top of another. There are seven bones (C1–C7) in the neck region. At the back of each vertebrae is an arch of bone that is designed to protect the spinal cord as it travels down the cervical spine to the rest of the body (Fig. 1ab).
- The cervical spine nerves come off the spinal cord and travel through holes in the side of the bone (transverse foramen) before traveling to the shoulder region and upper extremity (Fig. 1ab).
- In between the vertebrae are discs composed mostly of water and cartilage. The discs consist of an outer layer, called the annulus fibrosus, and an inner layer, called the nucleus pulposus. The outer layer is composed of alternating layers of cartilage (similar to your car tires) that

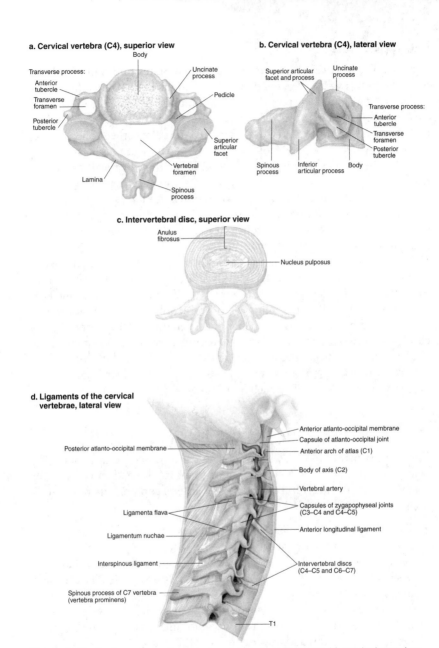

a. Cervical vertebra (C4), superior view

- Body
- Transverse process:
  - Anterior tubercle
  - Transverse foramen
  - Posterior tubercle
- Lamina
- Uncinate process
- Pedicle
- Superior articular facet
- Vertebral foramen
- Spinous process

b. Cervical vertebra (C4), lateral view

- Superior articular facet and process
- Uncinate process
- Transverse process:
  - Anterior tubercle
  - Transverse foramen
  - Posterior tubercle
- Spinous process
- Inferior articular process
- Body

c. Intervertebral disc, superior view

- Anulus fibrosus
- Nucleus pulposus

d. Ligaments of the cervical vertebrae, lateral view

- Posterior atlanto-occipital membrane
- Ligamenta flava
- Ligamentum nuchae
- Interspinous ligament
- Spinous process of C7 vertebra (vertebra prominens)
- Anterior atlanto-occipital membrane
- Capsule of atlanto-occipital joint
- Anterior arch of atlas (C1)
- Body of axis (C2)
- Vertebral artery
- Capsules of zygapophyseal joints (C3–C4 and C4–C5)
- Anterior longitudinal ligament
- Intervertebral discs (C4–C5 and C6–C7)
- T1

Figure 1. Illustrations show a) cervical vertebra, superior view; b) cervical vertebra, lateral view; c) intervertebral disc, superior view; d) ligaments of the cervical vertebrae (lateral view). (From Tank PW, Gest TR. *Lippincott Williams & Wilkins Atlas of Anatomy.* Baltimore, MD: Lippincott Williams & Wilkins; 2009.)

provides strength when we twist and turn our neck. The inner layer is more like a jelly ball that helps lessen the forces to the neck when we bend and turn the head and neck region. As we age, the discs lose their water content and become stiffer. If a disc herniates, it will compress the spinal nerve near the intervertebral foramen leading to pain that radiates into the upper extremity (Fig. 1c).

- Ligaments around the vertebrae act like guide wires that assist in movement of the neck in multiple directions. The ligaments are broader in the front (anterior) of the spine than the back (posterior) of the spine near the spinal cord. The thinner posterior ligament covers less of the disc and is a potential area of weakness (Fig. 1d).

- Finally, there are multiple layers of muscles that provide additional support and assist with motion. Some muscles work over short distances to stabilize the various bones, whereas others work over longer distances to assist with rotation and bending of the spine. All of the structures must work in concert so you can turn your head sideways or up and down (Fig. 2).

Imaging

Various imaging modalities allow us to look at the structures of the neck when we are concerned about a serious injury. X-rays and CT scans are helpful in assessing bone alignment, arthritis, and fractures. In the normal standing position, the cervical vertebrae are slightly curved in a reverse "C" shape as shown in Figure 3a. With injury, the cervical spine may straighten due to an underlying fracture or muscle spasm (Fig. 3b). Excessive curvature of the cervical spine may occur with weak muscles or problems in other areas of the spine. Figure 4 shows a posture with the head pushed forward due to a hunch in the middle of the thoracic spine (kyphosis). Clearly, proper posture of the neck and back may help in preventing subsequent injury (Fig. 5).

An MRI is useful for assessing disc herniations, the spinal cord, the ligaments, and the surrounding bony structures. Figure 6a shows a normal MRI of the spine from the side view (sagittal), whereas Figure 6b shows a disc herniation. Caution should be taken in looking at MRI, as studies have shown that we develop abnormal images as we age, even though we may not have symptoms. As an example, for asymptomatic individuals older than the age of 40 years, 60% exhibit degenerative discs, 20% have narrowing around the area where the nerves exit the spine, and 5% have disc herniations, even though they have no pain. Twenty-five percent of individuals younger than the age of 40 years exhibits degenerative discs. So speak with your doctor to better understand whether the MRI findings fit with your symptoms.

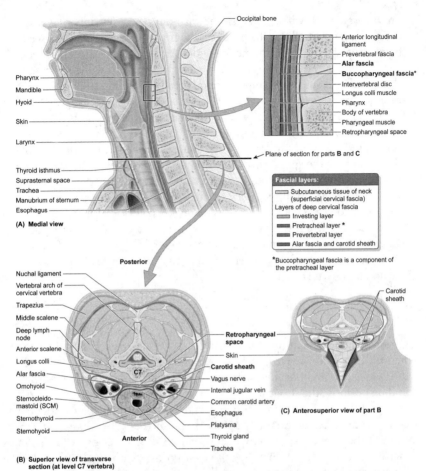

Figure 2. Muscles in the cervical spine. (From Moore KL, Agur AMR, Dalley AF. *Clinically Oriented Anatomy. 7th ed.* Baltimore, MD: Lippincott Williams & Wilkins; 2014.)

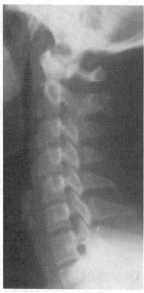

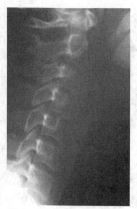

Figure 3b. Side view x-ray with a straightened cervical spine.

Figure 3a. Side view x-ray of the cervical spine.

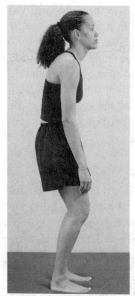

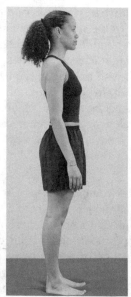

Figure 4. Excessive curvature of the neck with a hunched upper back.

Figure 5. Good posture of the spine.

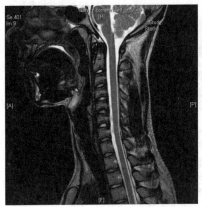

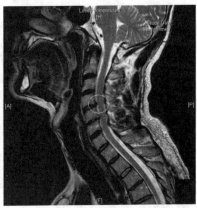

Figure 6a. Normal MRI of the cervical spine (side view).

Figure 6b. Abnormal MRI of the cervical spine showing a disc herniation.

Common Injuries and Disease of the Neck

Fortunately, the majority of injuries to the neck are due to muscle strains. Often, these injuries are due to nontraumatic mechanisms that may occur while performing an unfamiliar exercise or holding your neck in an unnatural position. Conservative treatment as outlined in the following text can quickly alleviate most of the symptoms related to muscle strains. Any neck pain that occurs due to trauma should be evaluated by a physician to assure there is no underlying fracture or injury to the spinal cord. In addition, neck pain associated with tingling in the hand or night pain should be evaluated by a physician. In these cases, a thorough history, physical examination, and special imaging may be required to determine the cause of your symptoms. The following are common causes of neck pain.

Acute Muscle Strain

Muscle strains are the most common cause of acute neck pain. These injuries typically occur during sudden, unexpected movement (i.e., quick rotation of the head while playing a sport/exercising) or slowly from poor posture during prolonged positions (i.e., bending over desk for hours, placing your computer too high/low, or sleeping in an uncomfortable position). The pain is described as achy to sharp in nature, involving the muscles around the back and side of the neck but not along the bony midline of the neck. Often, rotating the neck to the opposite side, stretching the involved injured muscle, worsens the pain. Although the pain may radiate to the head or shoulder, it is not usually associated with tingling involving the arm or hand. Coughing or sneezing does not typically worsen the pain. Pushing on the muscle and stretching of the muscle will reproduce the pain. The majority of acute neck muscle strains will usually resolve over a 6-week period with relative rest, avoidance of activities that exacerbate the symptoms, use of cold or heat packs, pain medication, or massage. A healthcare provider should evaluate symptoms lasting longer than the 6-week period. They may perform imaging to assess for other causes of neck pain and/or treat the symptoms with stronger pain medications, physical therapy, or injections.

Disc Herniation

Cervical disc herniations are less common—but potentially more serious—injuries to the neck. They occur in about 8 of every 1,000 persons and are most likely to occur in individuals age 50 to 54 years. A disc herniation occurs when the inner substance of the disc (nucleus pulposus) ruptures through the outer layer of the disc (annulus fibrosus), causing inflammation and compression of the nerves of the neck. (Picture jelly coming out of a jelly donut [Fig. 7].) The inflammation is from chemicals that are released during the herniation, whereas compression occurs from the inner disc substance pushing on a nerve. A disc herniation may occur when performing lifting activities or turning the head with the chin down toward the chest (flexion). Patients typically complain of sharp pain involving the region of the neck with radiation of the pain to the arm or hand. They may note tingling involving the arm or hand in a specific area. The symptoms are worsened with bending the neck forward and/or rotating the neck to the same side as the symptoms in the arm. Coughing or sneezing will often make the symptoms worse. Anyone experiencing a potential disc herniation should seek a proper evaluation by a physician. Treatment can range from

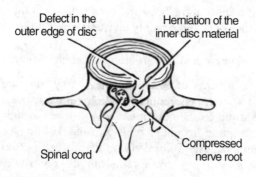

Horizontal Section
Figure 7. Lumbar disc herniation.

the use of medication, physical therapy, injections, and surgery, depending on the extent of the symptoms.

Arthritis

Many of us get arthritis of the spine over time. However, not everyone has pain related to arthritis of the neck. Arthritis occurs with increasing age as the cartilage wears away and the space between the bones narrows. Cervical spine arthritis is quite uncommon in individuals younger than the age of 40 years. In the neck, arthritis is associated with a loss in the height of the disc and overgrowth of the bone, which may narrow space for your nerves. Pain due to arthritis of the spine is gradual in onset, slowly occurring over weeks, months, or years. The pain is described as dull in nature and worsened with any movement of the neck. The pain may radiate toward the shoulder region but is not associated with tingling in the hand unless the bony narrowing impinges a nerve. Often, patients report neck stiffness upon arising in the morning and lessening of the pain during the day with continued motion. Treatments include activity modification, pain medication, and exercise (stretching and strengthening). Arthritis that develops into significant narrowing of the spine may lead to loss of function of the extremities and/or balance issues. Therefore, it is important to seek an evaluation by your healthcare provider if you notice any of these symptoms.

Preventive Measures

As noted before, a neck strain may occur due to performing an unfamiliar exercise or holding your neck in an unnatural position. Two common positions that lead to subsequent neck strain include

1. The "forward-thrust" position of the head and neck with resultant excessive curvature of the spine and possibly unusual stress on the neck muscle (Fig. 4).
2. Holding the neck rotated or twisted for a prolonged period of time.

Patients may find themselves in either of these positions during common daily activities. Any task in which the head and neck are extended and bent over work may cause strain to the neck muscles. Examples include working at a desk or on a computer, reading a tablet, sewing, knitting, or talking on the phone without a headset. Bifocal glasses that force a person to tilt his or her head while performing certain tasks can also contribute to neck strains. Even resting can cause neck strain if the patient does it in an improper position. Reading while propped in bed, watching television while stretching on a sofa, or sleeping in bed with a pillow that is too high are frequent causes of neck strains. Sleeping in a chair without proper posture or neck support should be avoided.

Figures 8 through 21 illustrate unnatural body positions that are common causes of neck strains during everyday activities. In addition, the figures note the proper positions to help prevent such injury. If your neck pain impacts your ability to perform your job, you should consider a "work-site evaluation" to assure the proper placement of work equipment, such as the computer, to help prevent subsequent injury.

Tips:
- Keep your neck drawn back, your chin comfortably tucked in, your shoulders relaxed, and your lower back straight while sitting (Figs. 8 and 9).
- Use a chair with support of the back to prevent your head and neck from being thrust forward (Figs. 8 and 9).

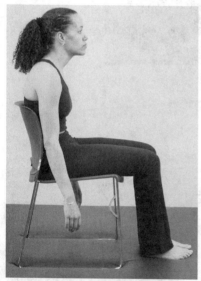

Figure 8. Don't slouch forward with rounded shoulders while sitting in a chair.

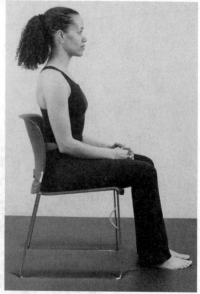

Figure 9. Proper posture for sitting in a chair.

- Make sure your chair is the right height, neither too low nor too high. Sit straight and avoid having to stretch forward or backward while working, eating, and so forth (Figs. 10 and 11).

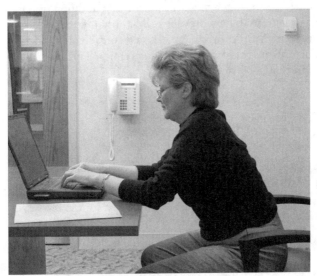

Figure 10. Don't lean away from your desk.

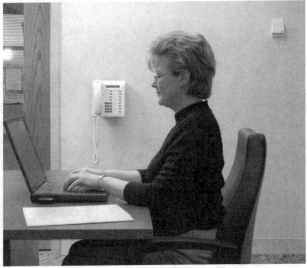

Figure 11. Proper posture for working at a desk.

- Keep your back and neck straight with your head level while reading (Figs. 12 and 13).

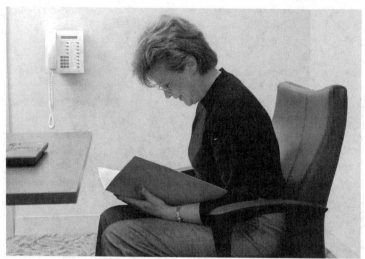

Figure 12. Don't bend your head too far down while reading.

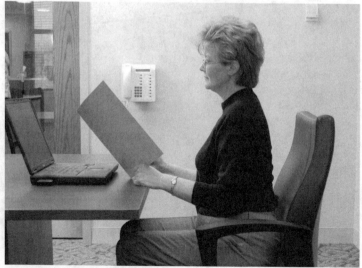

Figure 13. Proper posture while reading.

- Make sure your computer and keyboard are at a proper height and in a straight line to prevent twisting of the neck (Figs. 14 and 15).

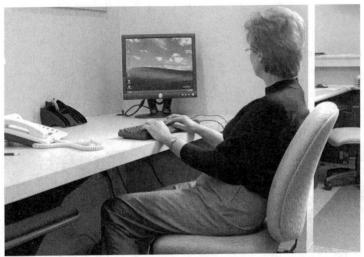

Figure 14. Don't twist your neck or head while working on a computer.

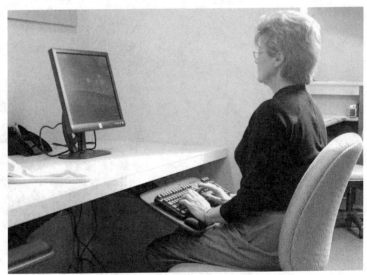

Figure 15. Proper alignment of body and computer.

- Use a headset while talking on the phone (Figs. 16 and 17).

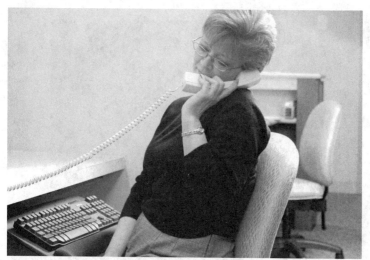

Figure 16. Don't twist your neck to hold the phone.

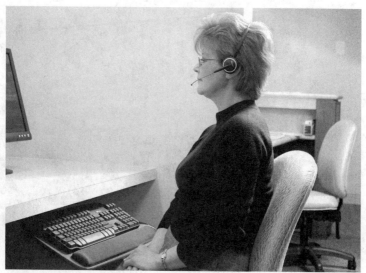

Figure 17. Proper use of headset to avoid neck pain.

- Make sure your car seat is adjusted properly. If it is too far forward or too low, you will need to stretch your neck forward to see (Figs. 18 and 19).

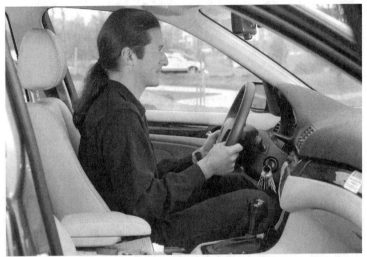

Figure 18. Don't drive with the seat too far forward.

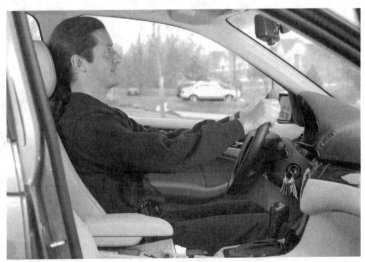

Figure 19. Proper posture while driving a car.

- If you are reading on a bed, sit with the proper support to rest your neck. Consider resting your arms on a pillow (Figs. 20 and 21).

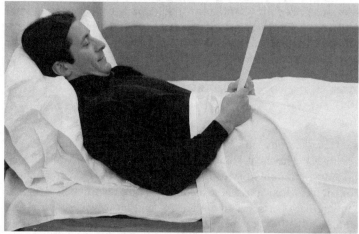

Figure 20. Don't slouch while reading in bed.

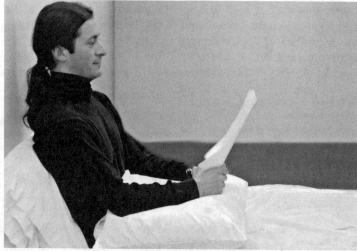

Figure 21. Proper posture while reading in bed.

Treatment Options

Proper treatment of any neck injury requires supervision by a physician, especially when there is trauma to the neck, prolonged pain, or associated tingling involving the arm. Fortunately, patients have a variety of options to treat less serious neck pain symptoms. A patient may consider trying some of these basic options prior to seeking medical attention. However, the patient should be sure to discuss with a physician any treatments and obtain the physician's approval before progressing with any exercises, especially if they worsen neck pain.

Medication

A variety of medications may be used to relieve the pain symptoms and improve recovery. The most common medications are called NSAIDs or nonsteroidal anti-inflammatory drugs. Common NSAIDs include ibuprofen, naproxen, or meloxicam. These medications are helpful in treating the pain and inflammation associated with neck pain. However, potential side effects include acid reflux, stomach ulcers, and problems with your kidneys. The patient should always discuss the use of any medication with his or her physician to ensure that there are no issues preventing the use of such medications in treating the pain. Acetaminophen is another common medication that may be used to help with pain relief. It has fewer side effects and is gentler on the stomach but should be used cautiously in anyone who has liver disease. Topical creams such as BenGay or IcyHot may provide symptomatic relief of pain as well. Other medications such as narcotics, muscle relaxers, or tramadol should only be used under the supervision of a physician.

Modalities and Bracing

Modalities include the application of such interventions as ice, heat, electrical stimulation, or ultrasound to the muscles of the neck. Several of these modalities may be applied by the patient. Others require a licensed professional trained in its proper use.

- *Ice:* After acute injury, you should use ice for any muscle pain to reduce pain and swelling. Ice is the preferred modality to be used intermittently for the first 48 hours following an injury. Although, it may be used longer if you find it is helping your symptoms. Cold packs, frozen vegetable packs, or ice bags can be used. Ice packs should be wrapped in a cloth or towel so that they are not placed directly on the skin. Direct application to skin can be uncomfortable and cause damage to skin. Ice packs are most helpful if used several times a day for approximately 10 to 15 minutes.

- *Heat:* Heat helps relieve pain and promotes circulation and muscle relaxation. Heating packs, electric heating pads, or moist-heated towels can be used. Moist heat, as applied through a hot pack or warm towel, should be applied to the involved area to help relax your muscles prior to performing gentle stretching exercises. Heat should be used cautiously in the first 48 hours because it may increase the amount of inflammation and swelling. Heat packs should be wrapped in a cloth or towel so that they are not placed directly on the skin. Direct application to skin can be uncomfortable and burn the skin.
- *Ultrasound:* This modality utilizes heat and ultrasound waves to treat your muscle pain. Ultrasound treatment should only be applied by a professional trained in its proper use.
- *Electrical stimulation:* Electrical stimulation as applied through E-Stim or a TENS unit can assist with the reduction of pain. Similar to the use of ultrasound, the treatment should only be applied by a professional trained in its proper use.
- *Massage:* Gentle massage, consisting of kneading or stroking of the neck muscles, can help alleviate some pain. However, massage is most effective when administered by a licensed professional massage therapist.
- *Neck brace:* At times, some physicians will prescribe a neck brace to relieve some of the stress to the muscles of your neck. However, you should not use the neck brace for more than a few days because prolonged use will lead to deconditioning of the neck muscles and worsening pain.

Physical Therapy

For more severe pain, a physician may prescribe physical therapy to treat neck pain symptoms depending on the cause of the pain. Physical therapists will utilize a variety of the modalities listed earlier to decrease the pain and increase the neck's range of motion. The patient will then progress to a series of neck stretching and strengthening exercises. These exercises are listed in the following text and should be incorporated into a home exercise program. It is extremely important to perform your exercises on a daily basis to assist in recovery and prevent deconditioning of the muscles of the neck.

Injections

Injection techniques may include interventions such as acupuncture, trigger point injections, or injections into the spine. Chronic muscle pains may respond to acupuncture or trigger point injections. In theory, they assist in relaxing the muscle by inhibiting an area of spasm. Interventional spinal procedures may include injections to the spinal nerves (epidural or transforaminal) if there is a disc herniation or joints (facets) if the pain is due to arthritis. A specially trained practitioner should only perform these procedures.

Exercises

The following series of exercises is specifically designed to stretch and strengthen the muscles in the neck. If the patient is recovering from a neck strain or have chronic neck stiffness, he or she should start the exercises slowly and gradually build up your strength and endurance until you can perform them several times per day. Mild increased soreness or stiffness may occur the day after performing these exercises. However, prolonged or worsening pain should lead to an evaluation by a physician. The patient should discuss the exercise program with a doctor before he or she begins and keep the doctor informed of the progress and any problems or questions. These exercises should be incorporated into a general exercise program that includes aerobic conditioning, such as walking, running, or cycling.

Stretching

The following stretches are designed to help increase the neck's range of motion. The patient should hold each stretch for 20 to 30 seconds and repeat each stretch two to three times, at least once a day. The patient should stretch the muscle until he or she feels a slight pull, but no further.

Exercise 1: Stretching of the neck muscles: sitting or standing. Place your right hand on the top of the head while your left hand grabs the seat of the chair or rests at your side. Using your right hand, gently pull the head toward the right to stretch the left neck muscles (Fig. 22). Hold for 20 to 30 seconds and relax. Repeat two to three times. Switch your hands and pull toward the left to stretch the right neck muscles.

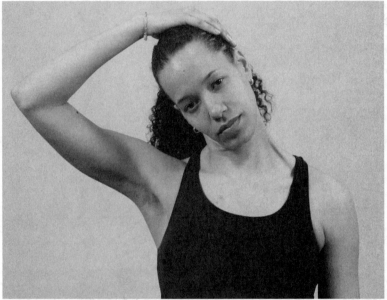

Figure 22. Stretching of the neck muscles.

Exercise 2: Stretching of the chest muscles: standing. Stand next to a wall. Place your right forearm on the wall with your elbow bent 90 degrees. Gently twist your upper body away to stretch the right chest muscles (Fig. 23). Hold for 20 to 30 seconds and relax. Repeat two to three times. Switch sides to stretch the left chest muscles.

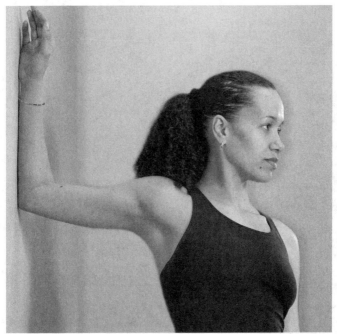

Figure 23. Stretching of the chest muscles.

Strengthening

After the pain has decreased and the range of motion has improved, the patient may gradually start strengthening exercise program. These isometric neck exercises are designed to increase the overall strength and stamina. The patient should hold each position for approximately 3 to 5 seconds and relax. Repeat each exercise three to five times as tolerated. Be sure to breathe properly throughout the exercises. For individuals under the guidance of a physical therapist or personal trainer, more complex strengthening exercises will be combined with functional exercises to promote a safe and speedy return to sporting activity.

Exercise 1: Chin tuck. Start with your head and neck in a normal posture (Fig. 24a). Gently pull your chin toward your chest as if you were nodding to someone (Fig. 24b). Hold for 5 seconds and return to your normal posture.

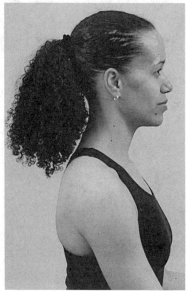

Figure 24a. Chin tuck—start position.

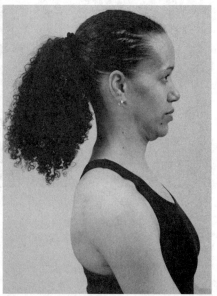

Figure 24b. Chin tuck—strength position.

Exercise 2: Isometric cervical retraction. Start with your head and neck in a normal posture. Place both hands onto the back of your head, intertwining the fingers. Push the head backward while resisting with the palms of your hands (Fig. 25). Hold for 5 seconds and relax.

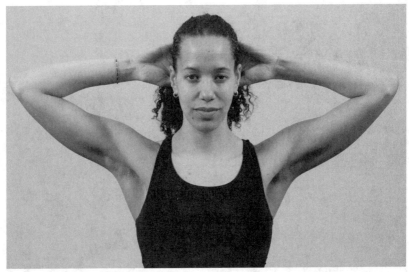

Figure 25. Resisted isometric cervical retraction.

Exercise 3: Isometric cervical rotation. Start with your head and neck in a normal posture. Place the palm of your left hand on the left side of your chin. Gently rotate your chin to the left while resisting with the palm of your left hand (Fig. 26). Hold for 5 seconds and relax. Repeat using the right hand and the right side of your chin.

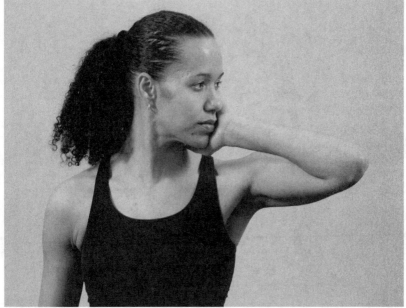

Figure 26. Resisted isometric cervical rotation.

Exercise 4: Isometric cervical side bending. Start with your head and neck in a normal posture. Place the palm of your left hand onto the left side of your head. Gently push your head to the left while resisting with your left hand (Fig. 27). Hold for 3 to 5 seconds and relax. Repeat using the right hand and the right side of your head.

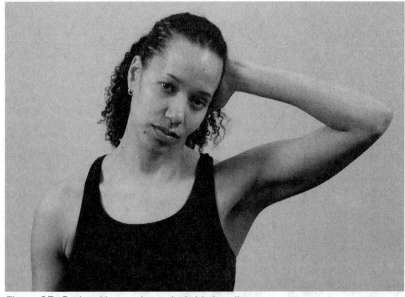

Figure 27. Resisted isometric cervical side bending.

Exercise 5: Isometric shoulder retraction. Start with your head and neck in a normal posture. You may consider clasping your hands behind your back if this action does not cause pain. Attempt to squeeze both of your shoulder blades together (Fig. 28a). Hold for 3 to 5 seconds and relax. Make sure you do not shrug your shoulders (Fig. 28b).

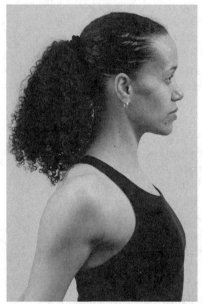

Figure 28a. Shoulder retraction—correct.

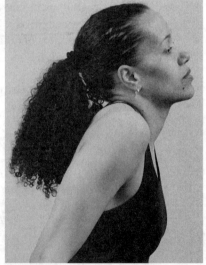

Figure 28b. Shoulder retraction—incorrect.

Summary

1. Neck pain is often due to muscle strains, which can be treated by proper rest, activity modification, medication, and exercises to improve posture. Severe neck pain or stiffness that does not respond to the earlier interventions could indicate a more serious problem that requires medical attention.

2. Attempt to avoid the habit of sitting with your head and neck thrust too far forward. Learn to stand and sit properly. This is especially important if a job puts the patient in a position that causes strain to the neck for a prolonged period of time.

3. Do not slump or slouch in unnatural positions while performing daily activities, such as lying on a sofa while watching television or reading while propped in bed.

4. Be sure to get enough rest. Stress and tiredness can contribute to the neck pain symptoms.

5. Exercise to stretch and strengthen the muscles in the neck. The patient should perform these exercises several times per week to maintain proper flexibility and strength.

6. The patient should incorporate neck exercises into a generalized exercise program including aerobic conditioning.

7. Maintain a healthy weight, as obesity may place increased pressure on the structures of your spine.

8. Eat a healthy, balanced diet to maintain good bone and muscle structure.

9. Do not smoke, as smoking has been associated with degeneration of discs.

Notes